MR. JONES' A

When it appears below, this book will have become a valuable first edition and your heirs will forever honor your memory!

MEDICARE
FOR THE LAZY MAN

SIMPLEST & EASIEST GUIDE EVER!

2021

Copyright 2020 Douglas B. Jones, CLU, RHU

This book and the content herein have been written in order to educate and to simplify a complex subject. Every effort has been made to ensure the accuracy of the content, but there is always room for misunderstanding and misinterpretation. Therefore, no liability is assumed for losses or damages due to the information provided.

The reader is responsible for his own choices, actions and results. He should seek guidance from professionals whenever there is any question as to the advisability of a particular course of action.

WHAT READERS SAY:

<u>Just what I needed</u>

As I get closer to the age when I have to decide on Medicare options, this book served as a great place to start. I also take comfort in the fact that, if I run across something I don't understand, I feel as though I can reach out to the author. I have even started listening to the podcasts - yep, I see I have some catching up to do! Thank you for making things easier to understand about Medicare, and setting me on the right course, as I now realize I should avoid Advantage Plans!

~LD STUART

<u>Well worth the price</u>

Simple and concise, easy to read booklet anyone can understand. Whittles the supplemental plans down to a couple that are best for most people. There are helpful links including one to Doug's website where you can send him a question. He got back to me quickly with helpful information. The booklet is well worth the price.

~KATIE BELL

<u>Informative, Understandable, and Funny</u>

This handy book makes the whole Medicare Supplement challenge manageable. It's clever, insightful, and is helpful in overcoming "Medicare Anxiety". An easy read worth the price.

~SVEA DARNALL

<u>The North Star of Medicare help guides</u>

Navigating the Medicare system for me is like studying contract law at Harvard. Doug is a brilliant tutor, full of crucial info, patience, and (thank God) wit. You can find most of the answers you need here in the book; and for those that aren't there, you can contact Doug in person! An informative, delightful read. Conan, NYC

~CONAN McCARTY

<u>The best advice for the majority, but you have to read with a critical and open mind to "get it"</u>
....after boring myself to death reading a couple other books on the topic, I decided to give this a fair shot and am I glad I did. The author points out very clearly his recommendations do not apply to those who are unhealthy or barely making it and even suggests asking for a refund.
Now, right to the point, the recommendations are simply brilliant. Keep in mind what insurance is meant for, protection against disasters, and don't forget that. You want the best coverage for when you need it most and the recommendations given are simply the best options available for those not in bad health or on welfare. The author breaks it down so simply and the numbers make sense 100%.
I'm glad I found this book because I have a Guarantee Issue event and I'm getting rid of the so called advantage plan and going with the recommendations made in this book. They are the only ones that make sense. Shame on the agents who push Medicare advantage and don't even mention these ultimate plans.
~DON PISTO

THIS BOOK IS DEDICATED TO:
LAZY MEN and the LAZY LADIES who love them, too smart to waste time and energy on stupidity!

It was written expressly for Medicare eligible Americans who:

- Are <u>not</u> infirm, but want to ensure that **protections** are in place if infirmity strikes.

- Are <u>not</u> destitute, but intend to get **maximum value** from the money spent on Medicare coverages.

- Want to understand **cost effective** ways to defend against catastrophic financial impact of medical treatment.

- Most of all, seek a **simple and clear** explanation of Medicare in order to make the best possible choices.

Is it time to buy Medicare insurance?

Would you like me to assist you?

On the site below, go to the US map.

Click your state & answer very simple questions:

www.MedicareForTheLazyMan.com

(or email: DBJ@MLMMailbag.com)

There is never a charge for my professional advice.

Try out my podcast:

Medicare for the Lazy Man Podcast

Wherever fine podcasts are given away free of charge!

CONTENTS

INTRODUCTION

Welcome to the 2021 version of Medicare for the Lazy Man!

This is the fourth edition of a work that strives to make the reader's transition to Medicare a more pleasant one.

This massive Federal program was created back in the 1960s with the aim of helping older Americans cope with the rapidly rising cost of health insurance. A noble goal, but over the decades it has blown up into a complex and often confusing bureaucracy that can be frustrating to its intended beneficiaries.

Why does Medicare operate in a seemingly nonsensical way?

- The program has always been a political football.

- Government functionaries turn up their noses at the superior examples set by private industry; insurance companies have the expertise and motivation to perform the same functions better, cheaper and much more cheerfully.

- Some genius decided it would be a great idea to copy the very first health insurance plans ever created, back in the mist-shrouded dawn of history.

So, the government created its own insurance company. In the process it also laid the foundation for a pervasive myth that is subscribed to by many of the people approaching Medicare age.

The myth in question holds that:

1) Unless one learns about every little aspect of the program there is a risk of errors.

2) These errors will cause disaster and doom that will haunt one for the rest of one's miserable, wretched life.

I am here to reassure you that this is not true. There is no reason to fear the arrival of Medicare; it is likely to be a very positive change in your life.

In the Obamacare world of health insurance for those who are pre-Medicare, the available protection is usually skimpy and very expensive.

When I first learned about group medical insurance, a monthly premium of around $10 would buy coverage for a 30-39 year-old with a $500 deductible, an unlimited lifetime maximum and with no restrictive provider network of doctors and hospitals.

That kind of value is a thing of the past everywhere except under Medicare. Fortunately, politicians who caused disaster in the health insurance markets did not have the political courage to destroy this program that continues to provide a good benefit for the price its participants are charged.

So long as Medicare remains a political "third rail", those who enter its portals will discover that much of what they find in Medicare Land will be cause for celebration!

Those celebrants, by the way, comprise a very large and growing tribe. We Baby Boomers (born 1946 to 1964) are a population cohort that looks like a fat rat passing through a snake. There is a great deal of money to be earned by selling us insurance to protect against the gaps in Medicare coverage.

Normal people view Medicare as an impenetrable mass of complexities. Most who are approaching age 65 would very much like to avoid having to study and learn about health insurance but fear that would result in poor choices and a lifetime of misery.

There is one class of abnormal people who purport to have studied and memorized mountains of Medicare minutia. They expect to be referred to as "consultants", "advisors" and "experts". Of course they do!

In my view, many of them are just "leeches". They routinely troll for fresh victims who will buy their commission-rich Medicare Advantage products. The leeches will razzle-dazzle their targets with snake-oil salesmanship, resulting in an aging population that is burdened with inferior protection.

These people are licensed agents and we are forced to purchase through them because the states have mandated it so. The commissions to be earned from selling us Medicare-related insurance represent a substantial source of income for the insurance agent.

By now you may have realized that I am also a leech, a licensed agent. I also love to earn commission dollars and view my fellow Boomers with much fiscal lust in my heart. However, the advice I offer to my clients and readers has some major differences from what they will often receive from my fellow leeches.

My advice:

1) **is much shorter and easier to grasp**
2) **may offer a bigger bang from the bucks you spend.**
3) **allows you to tell your agent exactly what you intend to purchase (and why).**

Studying all of the minutia about Medicare is going to be a huge waste of time and effort... unless you enjoy that sort of thing, of course.

Why? Because knowledge does NOT equal power! Nothing you memorize about Medicare will allow you to improve it in order to get better or cheaper protection. Also, any implication that disaster will ensue if your Medicare choices are not absolutely perfect is equally false.

In reality, very few Medicare decisions are completely irrevocable; mistakes and poor choices can often be fixed within a year or less.

Generally, the costliest mistakes actually stem from refusal to act, as in the case of late enrollment penalties. Later on, I provide a step-by-step guide to Medicare enrollment and the acquisition of related insurance that will complete the process for the majority of readers in average circumstances.

Look for **"The only chapter you are likely to need"** near the end of this book for a synopsis of my recommendations.

NOMENCLATURE: <u>PARTS</u> vs. <u>PLANS</u>

Original Medicare consisted of two elements called **<u>PARTS</u>:**

PART A – *covers inpatient treatment in a hospital or skilled nursing facility, hospice and home health care*

PART B – *covers outpatient treatment in doctors' offices, etc.*

<u>Added to the Medicare program more recently are:</u>

PART C – *So called "Advantage Plans" which I do not recommend*

PART D – *Prescription Drug Plans (PDP) defray the cost of drugs*

<u>Coverages that supplement Medicare are called **PLANS**:</u>

MEDICARE SUPPLEMENT <u>PLANS</u> – *protect against the gaps in Medicare*

PRESCRIPTION DRUG <u>PLANS</u> – *PDPs which defray the cost of drugs*

<u>IN THIS BOOK I ONLY DISCUSS</u>:

MEDICARE <u>PART A</u>

MEDICARE <u>PART B</u>

MEDICARE SUPPLEMENT <u>PLANS</u>

PRESCRIPTION DRUG <u>PLANS</u>

<u>These four provide the best protection available.</u>

CHAPTER 1

What sane person wants to read this stuff?

Why have you decided to buy *(or shoplift?)* this book?

- Are you closing in on Medicare age?
- Leaving job-related group insurance?
- Responsible for advising a friend or relative?
- Reexamining choices you made in the past?
- Suffering from insomnia?
- Paying the price for a dissolute life?

Are you seeking a quick roadmap through the Medicare maze?

What is your destination?

Until I dragged her out west to the University of Arizona, my wife attended a Catholic grade school and Jr. High, a Catholic girl's academy and a Catholic women's college.

Eventually I realized that Catholic schools do not teach geography because she cannot navigate her way out of a wet paper bag.

However, if you treat this book like a map and follow my suggestions, you will be able to easily navigate to your goal of selecting and acquiring the essential layers of coverage necessary for protection under Medicare:

MEDICARE PART A

MEDICARE PART B

MEDICARE SUPPLEMENT PLANS

PRESCRIPTION DRUG PLANS

That is all you need for complete protection, and it is very likely that these coverages will serve you well for the many decades of life you have yet to enjoy.

There will be no need to do an annual review or renewal for anything except perhaps the Prescription Drug Plan (PDP) and then only if you want to make sure yours is the least costly plan available.

Aiming to simplify a complex subject.

If that simplification is successful it should relieve the angst many feel when the time comes to make decisions about Medicare coverage.

Overall, there are three groups of people that may benefit most by considering the recommendations they will find here:

1) Those aged 64 who are preparing for initial Medicare enrollment.
2) Those aged 65 or older who are planning to leave their current employer sponsored insurance plan.
3) Existing Medicare participants who want to consider improving the quality or cost of their coverage.

Among these pages the average citizen confronting Medicare for the first time will discover a short, direct path from start to finish that will relieve their concerns and likely save them some money.

Notice I said "average citizen". The recommendations in this book are not for everyone, but the target audience includes the majority of those approaching Medicare eligibility.

My book has been written for those with:

Average or better health
Average or better financial resources
No desire to waste time or effort studying Medicare

Most helped will be people responsible for their own health insurance, specifically those about to turn 65 and employed people contemplating retirement or termination from an employer's health insurance plan.

Those who are destitute or stricken with debilitating medical conditions should drop this book and seek advice from their state's Medicaid (welfare) office and/or insurance agents in their immediate locale. Most areas of the US have "special needs plans" locally available and designed specifically for people in dire straits.

Once again, if you are infirm or destitute, stop reading right now and try to get a refund. This book is not for you!

CHAPTER 2

WHAT THE HECK DOES MEDICARE DO?

If you spent some of the 1960s within range of WLS-AM 890, Chicago's 50,000-watt rock blowtorch, you probably heard the legend of a very lazy young guy named Hootie Sapperticker. DJ Art Roberts promoted June 22 as Hootie Sapperticker Day, but the campaign never really gained traction and Hootie eventually faded into obscurity.

Decades later, Hootie and the Mrs. turned age 65 and, with my guidance, signed up for Medicare through the government on its "oh so user-friendly" website.

Because they learned that Medicare coverage is full of gaps and flaws, they also purchased insurance to protect themselves from those weaknesses in the program - insurance to supplement Medicare known as a **Medicare supplement.** Clever, huh?

As luck would have it, Mr. & Mrs. Sapperticker have a cute little grandchild who spends part of every day in a bubbling germ factory called nursery school. After enjoying hugs and kisses from this grandchild, they each contracted a major dose of the most virulent flu of the season. Surviving this disease required visits to a hospital ER, laboratory testing and several follow-up appointments with the family doctor after being released from confinement.

Hooty Sapperticker expected massive medical bills to start arriving shortly after treatment, but that did not happen. Because they are protected by Medicare, the invoices from the hospital, the doctors, the laboratory etc. were all sent to the federal government for payment. That process started as the patients showed their ID cards to office staff when treatment began.

After calculating and paying their share, the government functionaries (in the guise of Medicare) sent notification to the insurance company that issued their Medicare Supplement policies. The clerks at the insurance company double-checked the government calculations and then issued payment to the providers of medical treatment for the balances due them.

Months after their full recovery, the financial consequences of their illness were resolved. The very conservative Mrs. Sapperticker had purchased the Cadillac of all Medicare supplement plans and paid a monthly premium of around $160. She was delighted to find that her medical bills were paid in full – 100% coverage.

On the other hand, Hooty has always been more of a risk-taking party animal. He had purchased the high-performance Pontiac GTO of Medicare supplement plans for about $50 per month. Hooty had to write checks for a few hundred dollars in cost sharing because of the deductible his plan carries, but this was more than offset by the $100+ he saves each month in lower premiums. In addition, his beer funds have been protected from bill collectors.

The happy conclusion is that I, as the Sapperticker family insurance advisor, have been elevated to heroic status and toasted in absentia every time they gather together.

The cute little grandchild was never told about all of the misery caused by his grandparents' unconditional love.

SO, WHAT IS THE BIG DEAL ABOUT MEDICARE, ANYWAY?

Now that we understand **Medicare is a simple bill paying mechanism** for those Americans it covers, why is there such a hoo-rah about it?

Hapless citizens in their middle sixties are accosted with piles of insurance company propaganda and endless warnings about the dangers of charging into Medicare without professional guidance. Commission-driven leeches who promote themselves as "experts" are always happy to foster confusion that leaves customers vulnerable to their influence.

Other, more altruistic advisors have opined that responsible citizens must thoroughly read piles of insurance company propaganda, Medicare-related textbooks and other scholarly tomes. They have also suggested attending educational seminars and meeting with government officials in their offices. The implication is that you risk financial disaster and eternal damnation if you do not study and memorize all aspects of the Medicare morass.

This is a complete load!
It is really all about the commissions, folks!

This is why you will be buried in pitches for Medicare Advantage plans that have the richest commission schedules, followed by smaller piles of come-ons for Medicare Supplement plans that have less generous commission schedules by which insurance agents are paid.

However, you will never be told about my favorite plan, the best kept secret in Medicare. In order to force a discussion about the plan I most often recommend, you will have to grab the typical agent by the lapels and say the magic words: **high deductible.**

More about this closely guarded secret later in the book.

CHAPTER 3

Medicare Part A

Your goal in buying, borrowing or stealing this book should be to minimize the time and effort required to establish your Medicare related coverages. Let's get after it!

MEDICARE PART A is health insurance provided by the Federal government. It is intended to reimburse most of the expenses incurred during treatment in an inpatient facility (hospital, skilled nursing and rehabilitation) as well as hospice and limited home health care.

In almost all cases, Americans with a 10-year work history (or those married to someone with a 10-year history of taxable employment) will have Part A provided to them free of charge.

Since it is free, almost everyone is advised to enroll in Part A coincident with their 65th birthday (note the HSA exception below).

That coverage effective date (as with all Medicare-related coverages) will be on the first of the month in question.

Generally, someone turning 65 may enroll up to three months before the birthday month begins. Coverage will then go into effect on the 1st day of that birthday month. They also have a few months available to enroll after the birth month, but this might mean going without coverage for some period.

Exception: if the actual date of birth is on the 1st of any month, coverages will become effective on the 1st day of the prior month.

Don't ask why this is so; nobody knows.

Exception: if the existing health insurance plan is an HSA (Health Savings Account) and you would like to continue making pre-tax contributions, regulations prohibit enrollment in any part of Medicare.

ENROLL IN MEDICARE PART A ONLINE HERE:
https://www.ssa.gov/medicare/

(**SSA** is the Social Security Administration, the government agency originally charged with overseeing the Medicare program.)

Scroll down to the blue button: Apply for Medicare Only

How To Apply Online For Just Medicare

If you are within three months of age 65 or older and not ready to start your monthly Social Security benefits yet, you can use our online retirement application to sign up just for Medicare and wait to apply for your retirement or spouses benefits later. It takes less than 10 minutes, and there are no forms to sign and usually no documentation is required.

Apply for Medicare Only

Return to Saved Application | Check Application Status | Replace Medicare Card

To find out what documents and information you need to apply, go to the Checklist For The Online Medicare, Retirement, and Spouses Application.

CHAPTER 4

Medicare Part B

At the risk of belaboring the obvious, the following is my official definition of the second part of Medicare:

MEDICARE PART B is health insurance provided by the Federal government. It is generally intended to reimburse expenses incurred during treatment by doctors, typically in an outpatient setting, as well as testing & diagnostics, medical equipment, supplies and preventive care.

It is important to choose the effective date of your Part B coverage very carefully. Medicare Part B carries a substantial monthly premium (starting at $148.50/month in 2021) so it would not be prudent to start it too early.

More important, since Medicare Part B is critically important protection designed to reimburse the costs of the most commonly encountered treatment, it would REALLY not be prudent to enroll too late.

Late enrollment in Part B, after becoming eligible, risks incurring hefty medical expenses without insurance protection. If one fails to enroll until after the eligibility period, the opportunity to enroll will be limited to a short period at the beginning of each following year and coverage will not become effective for several months after that.

In addition, substantially late enrollment in Part B subjects one to a lifetime monetary penalty that will be added to the monthly premium forever.

The importance of timely Part B enrollment cannot be stated too strongly.

Turning age 65:

Medicare eligible people who are responsible for their own health insurance will have no difficulty choosing an enrollment date. They will turn age 65 and will properly enroll with an effective date of the first day of their 65th birth month.

Exception: if the actual date of birth is on the 1st of any month, coverage will become effective on the 1st day of the **prior** month.

Don't ask why this is so; nobody knows.

The enrollment period begins 3 months before the birth month, and prudence dictates that the enrollment process should begin as early as practical within that 90-day period.

Retirement or departure from an employer's group medical plan after turning 65:

Medicare coverages should be scheduled to begin when the group plan terminates. It is not prudent to have any gap in coverage and it is really bad to have a gap lasting longer than 63 continuous days. At that point your medical history might come into play as to when you will be allowed to have full coverage for pre-existing medical conditions.

The enrollment application used for Medicare Part B is: CMS-40B and may be downloaded from numerous locations, including MedicareForTheLazyMan.com. It will be important to confirm that there was health insurance coverage in place just prior to the requested Part B effective date.

The form used to verify this is CMS – L564. It may be downloaded from numerous locations in the internet, including MedicareForTheLazyMan.com.

During the current virus panic some enrollment rules have been liberalized so the employer's signature on the CMS-L564 is not currently required.

Other circumstances that might affect your coverage decisions:

- Do you have a spouse who is actively employed?
- Are you not a US citizen?
- Are you on COBRA or retiree medical coverage from an employer group plan?
- Are you eligible for Tricare or other VA coverage?
- Do you fall into another category that complicates things?

If any of the above apply, you may need professional advice about whether, or exactly when to begin Medicare Part B coverage. You should seek that advice from any of the unbiased sources I have listed in the following chapter.

ENROLL IN MEDICARE PART B ONLINE HERE:

https://www.ssa.gov/medicare/

(**SSA** is the Social Security Administration, the government agency originally charged with overseeing the Medicare program. They use the word "retirement" repeatedly to mean Social Security.)

Scroll down to this section just above the blue "Apply" button:

Should I Sign Up For Medical Insurance (Part B)?

With our online application, you can sign up for Medicare Part A (hospital insurance) and Part B (medical insurance). Because you must pay a premium for Part B coverage, you can turn it down.

If you're eligible at age 65, your initial enrollment period begins three months before your 65th birthday, includes the month you turn age 65, and ends three months after that birthday.

If you choose not to enroll in Medicare Part B and then decide to do so later, your coverage could be delayed and you may have to pay a higher monthly premium for as long as you have Part B. Your monthly premium will go up 10 percent for each 12-month period you were eligible for Part B, but didn't sign up for it, unless you qualify for a "Special Enrollment Period" (SEP).

If you don't enroll in Medicare Part B during your initial enrollment period, you have another chance each year to sign up during a "general enrollment period" from January 1 through March 31. Your coverage begins on July 1 of the year you enroll. Read our Medicare publication for more information.

If you have a Health Savings Account (HSA) or health insurance based on current employment, you may want to ask your personnel office or insurance company how signing up for Medicare will affect you.

If the online enrollment becomes problematic, I suggest calling the nearest office of the Social Security Administration to ask how they suggest you proceed with the enrollment process and the submission of the required documents.

It appears to me that there is a lack of consistency in how enrollments are being facilitated presently, so it is best to ask for instructions from those who will be in charge of the procedures.

CHAPTER 5

SOURCES OF INFORMATION

Here are some (theoretically) unbiased sources of information and advice on choosing the proper Medicare effective date for you/your spouse:

Choosing a Medigap Policy: A Guide to Health Insurance for People with Medicare:

https://www.medicare.gov/pubs/pdf/02110-medicare-medigap-guide.pdf

Helpful contacts in each state
www.Medicare.gov/contacts

SSA: The Social Security Administration (which administers the Medicare program)
https://www.ssa.gov/medicare/

Enrolling in Medicare Part A & Part B

https://www.medicare.gov/Pubs/pdf/**11036**-Enrolling-Medicare-Part-A-Part-B.pdf
CMS Product No. 11036

Medicare & You 2021:

https://www.medicare.gov/Pubs/pdf/10050-Medicare-and-You.pdf

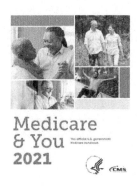

Medicare for Dummies Cheat Sheet

http://www.dummies.com/personal-finance/insurance/health-insurance/medicare-for-dummies-cheat-sheet/

SHIP – State Health Insurance Assistance Programs – choose your state from the drop-down menu
https://www.shiptacenter.org/

Public service agencies, like a local hospital for instance, may have a Medicare and Social Security advisor on staff.

Your company HR department

CHAPTER 6

Medicare Is Not Enough Protection!

If you have started the Medicare enrollment process with plenty of time to spare before the effective or starting date, of your coverage, take a break. Do something more fun or productive until confirmation of your successful enrollment arrives.

This confirmation could be in the form of a Medicare ID card received in the US mail, or a downloadable/printable card on your Medicare.gov account or a printable copy of their "benefits verification" letter.

Eventually, you will receive a Medicare ID card. It will show your unique alpha/numeric "identifier" and the start dates for Parts A and B.

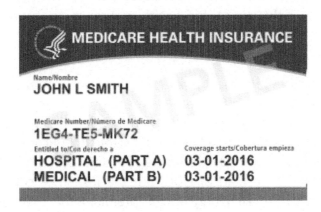

Now is the time to purchase the insurance that will protect you from the dangerous gaping holes in Medicare protection.

What are these gaping holes you ask? They are the deductibles, coinsurance, co-pays and unlimited lifetime cost sharing amounts that severely limit the protection afforded by original Medicare.

These cost sharing elements of Medicare Part A and Part B have no statutory limit. Potentially, very large amounts of money are at risk for people on Medicare who have not purchased additional protection from a private insurance company. Someone once calculated that, if everything that could go wrong did go wrong over $900,000 in medical expenses could be charged to a Medicare participant who was only covered by original Medicare.

Insurance to supplement Medicare

Two basic types of insurance are available to protect you from financial disaster. One is clearly superior.

1) **MEDICARE SUPPLEMENT PLANS** – The best and only choice for health insurance to supplement Medicare, assuming you can afford a modest monthly premium cost.

Medicare supplement plans range from very comprehensive to very cost effective. In keeping with my goal of simplification, I have only recommended the very richest Plan G or the streamlined High Deductible Plan G (HDG). People who turned 65 before 2020 (born before 1955) may select HDF instead of HDG, but the insurance companies seem to be ratcheting up the premiums on their regular Plans F so those are rapidly losing their allure.

If you are a youngster who first turned 65 in 2020 or later, the simplest and most comprehensive supplement plan available to you will be Plan G. The most cost-effective plan you will be allowed to purchase will be the brand-new High Deductible Plan G (HDG). These two plans operate just like their predecessors (F and HDF) except that they do not cover the Part B annual deductible, which is $203 during the year 2021.

MEDICARE SUPPLEMENTS GIVE YOU FREEDOM!

Read the next two chapters (7 & 8) to learn why I only recommend Medicare supplements to all of my clients.

2) **MEDICARE ADVANTAGE PLANS (PART C)** – Do not even consider these or waste your time learning about them.

This type of supplemental coverage actually removes Medicare Parts A & B, along with all of their benefits and protections. Original Medicare is replaced by an insurance company plan that forces participants into an HMO-like gulag of rules, regulations and restrictions. The only reason you hear about Medicare Advantage plans so often is that they pay very generous commissions to the insurance agent – thanks in large part to you, the American taxpayer.

You can read more about Medicare Advantage (Part C) in Chapter 9 if you have some time to kill.

CHAPTER 7

Medicare Supplement Plans:
The ONLY Way to Fly!

When compared with the highly-flawed Medicare Advantage (Part C) plans, Medicare supplement plans have only one disadvantage: they are not given away free of charge.

Each Medicare supplement plan has a monthly premium charge, although the costs vary widely between states, insurance carriers and type of plan.

The available plans are standardized from company to company and state to state. Each is denoted by a letter, so as an example, Plan A provides the same protections and benefits no matter which company sells it and no matter which state it is sold in.

In almost all states there are as many as twelve Medicare Supplement plans being sold, and they all have one great thing in common:

COMPLETE FREEDOM OF CHOICE!

1) Medicare supplement plans **never have restrictive networks of doctors and hospitals**.
   A person covered by a Medicare supplement plan is free to seek treatment from any provider anywhere who accepts Medicare patients. The greatest medical specialists in the world practice in various facilities around the United States and none of them have

been placed out of reach by an arbitrary insurance company network list enforcer.

2) No network means no **lists to consult when it comes to figuring out what providers to use, no risk of nasty surprises** when seeking treatment away from home or in an emergency situation.

3) A patient covered by a Medicare supplement may **seek treatment from any specialist anywhere without requesting permission** from a gate-keeper or primary care physician.

4) Medicare supplement plans, just like Medicare Parts A & B, are **good anywhere in the 50 US states and possessions**. The plans I recommend also have a $50,000 lifetime benefit for emergency treatment in foreign countries.

5) Medicare supplements are guaranteed renewable and will provide their benefits forever, just as long as premiums continue to be paid. The onset of critical illness will not cause the coverage to be changed or terminated. The insurance company must live up to all of its obligations but the policy holder's only obligation is to continue payments when due.

6) A cautionary note: After your initial period of guaranteed issue eligibility, insurance companies may question your medical history if you apply for a different plan or to a different company. My advice

is to choose your insurance carrier and your supplement plan very carefully because you just may have that plan for the rest of your life.

How does one decide which of the twelve Medicare supplement plans to purchase?

Follow my recommendation to buy either the luxurious Cadillac or the high-performance Pontiac of Medicare supplement plans.

LOTS OF BANG FOR REASONABLE BUCKS!

Two Medicare supplement plans I recommend for the average consumer:

The most comprehensive coverage allowed by law; **the luxurious Cadillac of Medicare supplements**:

PLAN G for those born in 1955 or later;

PLAN F for those who are older.

-OR -

Great protection at an exceedingly low price: **the high-performance Pontiac GTO of Medicare Supplements**:

HIGH DEDUCTIBLE PLAN G – for those born in 1955 or later; **HIGH DEDUCTIBLE PLAN F** for those who are older.

Each of these Medicare supplement plans covers **100%** of the following costs (except the Part B deductible as noted), filling in the many gaps in original Medicare:

Part A deductible
Part A coinsurance and hospital costs
(up to an additional 365 days after Medicare benefits
are used up)
Part A hospice care coinsurance or copayment

Part B deductible – NOT covered by Plan G
Part B coinsurance or copayment
Part B excess charges

Skilled nursing facility coinsurance

Blood (first 3 pints)

AND:

80% of foreign travel emergency expenses after a small
deductible
(up to a $50,000 lifetime total)

PLAN F has no deductibles, co-pays, co-insurance nor any
other cost sharing provisions. The insured person will not
receive any invoices for routine cost sharing expenses. You
cannot buy this plan if you were born in 1955 or after.

PLAN G will reimburse everything but the Part B deductible
($203 in 2021).

Plans HDF and **HDG** credit the above expenses to their
deductibles until they are met, and then pay at 100% for the
rest of the year.

Here is more about my favorite Medicare Supplement plans.
The simplest is **High Deductible Plan F**, which those born
before 1955 may continue to buy.

Newest is **High Deductible Plan G** which is available to
those born in 1955 or later. Its appearance confused some
experts but most agree that HDG credits all Medicare
eligible charges to its deductible with the exception of the
annual Part B deductible.

LET'S CALL THEM "HIGH VALUE PLANS"

Both of the high deductible plans are saddled with an unfortunate and scary name. The insured will NOT have to pay the first $2,370 of medical expenses, only the much smaller Part A or Part B deductibles, depending on the type of medical treatment they must have.

After that, if the treatment continues, Medicare pays the vast majority of the expenses while the High Deductible plan applies the smaller unpaid segment of the expenses to its deductible, leaving the practitioners to send invoices for those relatively small amounts to the insured.

The insured typically has been saving as much as $100 per month by not buying an expensive Plan F or G, so kicking in a few bucks here and there still leaves him with plenty of lettuce in his wallet.

Unless one is thrown into a hospital, these small invoices will be for 20% of the outpatient charges considered to be Medicare Part B expenses. Part B has an annual $203 deductible (in 2021) and then a 20% coinsurance for Part B treatment costs so individuals covered by the high deductible plans will pay 20% of their charges out-of-pocket in exchange for saving substantial premium dollars.

I illustrate in Chapter 8 that the term **"high deductible" is a complete misnomer**, since Medicare pays benefits no matter what supplement plan – if any – is in place.

This is why the term "**HIGH VALUE PLANS**" is much more accurate!

CHAPTER 8

The best kept secret in Medicare:
High Deductible "high value" plans!

High deductible plans are a terrific bargain! Too bad most agents won't talk about them. You see, they would rather earn hefty commissions than to give valuable advice that might cut into their earnings and save the client some money. The fact is, agents earn more when the product they sell is more costly!

The official description of these plans is that they have a hefty $2,370 "annual deductible" before picking up the balance of all unpaid medical bills. This completely ignores the fact that Medicare will begin paying the bills right after its very small deductible has been covered.

The insured **WILL NOT PAY THE FIRST $2,370 (in 2021)** of medical bills if they get sick or hurt! Medicare will pay the lion's share of the bills after the relatively small Part A/Part B deductibles (depending on the kind of treatment needed). The insured will pay a much smaller percentage of the bills until, in the unlikely event of a very bad year, his small portion adds up to the plan deductible. After that – 100% baby!

The name "high deductible" is completely misleading and the downside risk is so very limited that the average person will be flush with extra cash from the first month after buying the HD plan! The reality is that Medicare will have been paying 80% of outpatient expenses starting right after that $203 deductible!

This is why "HIGH VALUE" is a much better name!

Do you remember the beautiful days before Obamacare changed the health insurance landscape, driving up costs and removing many of the choices people could make? Most people had a medical plan that imposed a small deductible first, then a co-insurance or cost sharing period and finally began to pick up 100% of medical bills for the rest of the year.

For instance, a common plan could be described as having a $250 deductible, 80/20% co-insurance of the next $5000 and 100% thereafter. This was almost universal until a few years ago and did a good job of protecting people from otherwise painful medical bills.

A smart Medicare Supplement purchaser may keep a similar level of protection, and at a very small monthly premium charge. A person buying the High Deductible Plans F or G will have something like a $200 deductible, then 80/20% of the next $11,000 and then 100% coverage for the rest of the year.

MEDICARE WILL ALWAYS PAY ITS PORTION FIRST.

Medicare doesn't know whether there is a supplement or not, it just goes along paying its 80% of the outpatient bills (after the $203 deductible).

For Part A expenses, it pays all of the first 2 months of hospital charges after the $1,484 (per admission) deductible. This means Medicare pays 100% of hospital costs after a reasonable deductible and 80% coverage for outpatient expenses after a small deductible, even if there is no supplement in place. In the rare event of a disastrous series of medical events, the downside risk of High Deductible "high value" plans is very reasonable indeed.

As stated elsewhere, this book is written with a particular audience in mind: those who are not infirm and those who are not destitute. This group can generally afford to pay the reasonable price of regular Plans F or G, the Cadillac and most popular of Medicare supplement plans. However, as comprehensive as the benefits of F and G are, they may not be the most cost-effective choice.

My healthy clients always appreciate the cost/benefit of High Deductible (or **High Value**) plans once it is properly explained to them that the term "high deductible" is a complete misnomer. When we are talking about outpatient Part B expenses, what we really have is a $203 deductible and 20% coinsurance of the next $11,850. After that the plan pays 100% for the rest of the year.

It is extremely unlikely that the average person will have total bills anywhere near $12,000. That means he will be saving somewhere near $100 per month year after year by choosing a High Deductible **"High Value"** plan. So, in a good year, the policy owner will likely save $1200 or more in comparison to the higher cost of Plan F or even Plan G.

What if disaster strikes and medical expenses grow to a very large number in a given year? The insured person has plenty of downside protection from nasty surprises. If he has to spend all of that $2370 out of pocket towards the deductible and coinsurance, remember that he very likely saved $1200 in premium costs so that leaves just under $1200 (or about $100 per month on the average) to meet his share until the

High Deductible plan starts paying 100% for the rest of the year.

What about the monthly savings the insured enjoyed for the many years that expensive medical treatment was not needed? ...and what about the many years of good health and monthly savings that will follow that one unfortunate year?

MONEY IN THE BANK!

CHAPTER 9

Medicare Advantage (Part C) Plans: Why Not?

The only advantage I can see in Medicare Advantage plans is that they don't cost very much to buy. In fact, many of them have $0 monthly premiums! Good deal, right?

Sure, they can be a pretty good deal if nothing bad happens to you; no serious injury or illness that causes the need for medical treatment. In other words, you will be just fine with a Medicare Advantage plan until you actually need to use it.

Insurance agents love these plans because of the generous commissions they pay (thanks to the largess of the taxpayers). Why should you, the insurance buyer beware the hidden booby-traps in Medicare Advantage plans? Where are the flaws in Medicare Advantage or Part C plans for the potential customers like you?

The big one: **NO FREEDOM OF CHOICE!**

1) MEDICARE ADVANTAGE (Part C) plans are HMOs or PPOs. They all rely on networks of physicians and hospitals to deliver care. This adds the complication of having to choose your provider from a list of names to ensure treatment will be covered.

2) One must do comparison shopping every year because the networks are constantly in flux, with

some doctors quitting and others joining. If your favorite doctor were to quit your network, you would be stuck finding a replacement from the list given to you by the insurance company. Plans that include drug coverage will often change their formularies, sometimes rendering the whole plan a great deal more expensive.

3) The average Advantage plan has an out-of-pocket limit of over $5000 per year with some having a limit as high as $7500. Why would anyone be uncomfortable with a Medicare Supplement High Deductible (**High Value**) plan out-of-pocket limit of $2370 by comparison to that much higher possible loss?

4) Even the most highly touted Advantage plans can beat an insured to death with hidden fees and co-pays. One best selling plan in Florida has co-pays like this: ambulance: $300; hospital stay: $175 per day for first 10 days; diabetic supplies: 20% coinsurance; diagnostic radiology: up to $125 co-pay; lab services: $100 per day; outpatient X-rays: up to $100 per day; therapeutic radiology: $35 up to 20% co-pay; renal dialysis: 20% of the actual fee.

5) Costly complications can spring out of the bushes to cause unpleasant surprises. For example, your surgeon might belong to the network but the anesthesiologist he uses may not; the radiologist may be in the network but the specialists who interpret the films may not be. In these examples, you should expect to receive a hefty invoice in the mail.

6) Frequently, permission is required prior to seeking consultation with a specialist.

A lengthy investigation by the Inspector General of the department of HHS recently caught a number of these plans denying requests of this nature to all subscribers and then rolling over to change that decision for the small minority who displayed the moxie to file grievances. The other suffering members? I guess they either went without treatment or paid out-of-pocket.

7) Networks usually operate in a localized area and traveling out of it or living in a second home somewhere can be a problem, if medical treatment is needed.

8) They will promise that out-of-network emergency care is covered, but may balk at cooperating when it comes to paying for it.

9) Insurance agents who try to enroll hapless victims into a "low cost" or "free" Advantage plan will then sometimes badger them to purchase additional Hospital Indemnity insurance to pay the hidden expenses not covered by the Advantage plan.

10) The many extras they tout, like dental, vision and hearing coverage are often disappointing limited benefit discount plans rather than true insurance coverage. In addition, they rely on small networks of doctors and dentist, further restricting freedom of choice.

SOMETIMES WE GET WHAT WE PAY FOR!

How can an insurance company give away a product for free? This only works if the government pays the freight. When the government decides to cut its expenses, the insured clients will be the ones to pick up the slack. In the meantime, very large commissions mean that you will never cease hearing about the wonderful world of Medicare Advantage from insurance agents.

The good news is that holders of Medicare Advantage (Part C) plans are allowed to switch from one plan or company to another every year during AEP or Open Enrollment, which allows dissatisfied subscribers to try out a new plan to be effective the following January 1st.

Have you noticed that there is a huge amount of direct mail, TV ads, internet pop-ups and other annoying insurance talk happening every fall? This is because the poor saps who found themselves stuck with Medicare Advantage plans have an opportunity to try a different MA plan.... anything else to replace the crapola they bought last year.

Once again, **I do not recommend these plans** for my audience of Medicare eligibles who are not destitute or infirm.

CHAPTER 10

MEDICARE MSA:

An Advantage plan I actually like!

Freedom of choice is rare in the Medicare Advantage world, but I recently found an MA plan that might just cure that problem!

The standard MA (Part C) plans that flood your mailbox and assault your eyeballs often advertise themselves to be free of charge or have $0 premium. How do you think an insurance plan is able to assume the risk that an older person will need expensive medical treatment without charging a premium each month?

The answer? They receive cash directly from the government.

They use this money to pay medical providers, provide cheapo dental and vision coverage plus pretend to offer a bunch of other stuff to get people interested in signing up for eventual disappointment.

How do we know there is likely to be disappointment? Just look at the frenzied level of activity every October to December when all of these poor saps have an opportunity to dump their plan and try a different one.

Turns out 53 days in each fall wasn't long enough to satisfy the demand for freedom so the period has been extended into the new year, probably to avoid the risk of armed insurrection.

I have seen a glimmer of light on the horizon! It just might prove to be salvation for the Medicare Advantage industry.

It is a very dim light so far, but hope springs eternal!

The newly arrived product is a **Medicare MSA or "Medical Savings Account"** and it offers some of the best of both worlds: Advantage and Supplement in such a way that I can almost bring myself to recommend it.

The only thing stopping me from enthusiastic endorsement is the caution one feels after having seen so many high hopes dashed over the years.

The one Medicare MSA company with which I am most familiar is indeed offering a Medicare Advantage plan in the sense that its funds come from the government.

However, instead of keeping all that money while offering worthless baubles and empty promises to potential subscribers, this MSA actually gives a chunk of the funding directly to the subscriber. By "chunk" I mean thousands and thousands of US greenbacks.

This is the way one MSA plan works:

Medicare (the US government) gives the plan an infusion of funds; the plan then deposits some cash into a bank account in your name. It uses some of the rest to purchase a high deductible health insurance policy that pays 100% after the deductible. The balance of their funds is used for agent's commission, operating revenue and profit.

Here is what you, the purchaser of the plan will see:

1) A $0 premium Medicare Advantage plan with no restrictive network of doctors and hospitals. Any provider that accepts Medicare payment can be consulted anytime the patient chooses.

2) An annual deposit of either $2,000 or $3,000 (your choice) into a bank account in your name. How you spend, save or invest this money is entirely up to you.

3) A high deductible insurance policy will provide a ceiling on the amount at risk in the event of catastrophic medical expenses. The deductible will either be $5,000 or $8,000 for the year, depending on the amount of annual deposit for which you signed up.

4) The opportunity to roll over that deposit to the following year when another deposit will be made to your account, or withdraw the remaining funds in the account, pay income taxes and splurge on the rest.

5) The need to purchase the Prescription Drug Plan of your choice (as little as $7.00 in some areas in 2021).

My understanding is that several companies offer Medicare MSAs in their local regions. I only know of one company that operates in a multi-state, almost nationwide environment.

Until there is a demonstrated level of performance and stability, I am reluctant to broadly endorse the concept or the only Medicare MSA carrier I am contracted with.

If you want to take a closer look at this health insurance plan with a savings account component and an element of risk, contact me at my podcast e-mail address and I will send you a brochure: DBJ@MLMmailbag.com.

Freedom is a great thing; cross your fingers that it spreads across the land and defeats the evil Advantage monster!

CHAPTER 11

Drugs? We Don't Need No Stinkin' Drugs!

PDP, Prescription Drug Plan or Part D – buy it ASAP!

In their infinite generosity, the Feds now subsidize the cost of prescription drug plans that can be purchased from private insurance companies. Each of these companies can price their drug plans where they want to, compile their own list of drugs to be covered (formularies) and offer different levels of benefit to their customers.

Here are the problems: the construction of each drug plan sounds very complicated to the non-insurance professional; there are deductibles, co-pays, co-insurance and a big scary donut hole to contend with.

Additionally, the formularies and premiums can change from one year to the next and each individual's prescription medication requirements can change.

Therefore, I recommend comparing all available plans only on the basis of the estimated out of pocket cost per year. If the changes in formulary, premium cost or drug needs warrant, the insured can select a new company and a new plan during the annual open enrollment period for the following year.

There is a fairly painless way to compare the cost of all of the drug plans in your locality via the government website. Look for the easy navigation directions below.

What if you are so healthy that you take no prescription drugs at all? After thanking the ancestors who passed down your particular gene pool, consider whether there might be a need for insuring against high prescription costs anytime in the future. If not, and you expect to never, ever purchase one of these drug plans, you are finished right now.

On the other hand, most people without crystal balls like to keep their options open and hedge their bets. And they generally want to avoid the lifetime late enrollment penalty.

If a person becomes eligible to purchase a PDP but elects not to do that, and then decides to go ahead and buy one sometime in the future, a late enrollment penalty will be assessed for each month elapsed from the initial eligibility period to the actual purchase.

The penalty amounts to roughly 35 cents per month for each month elapsed. That means an extra $4.20 per month for a one-year delay, $8.40 per month for a two-year delay, $12.60 per month for a three-year delay and so on.

This is why I advise my clients to buy an inexpensive PDP (maybe $7.30 per month) when they are first eligible, even if they take no drugs yet.

Admittedly, not all have followed my advice, but I sleep better at night knowing that I tried.

Kind of like child rearing.

EASY NAVIGATION INSTRUCTIONS TO SELECT THE LOWEST COST PDP:

Go to site: https://www.medicare.gov/plan-compare

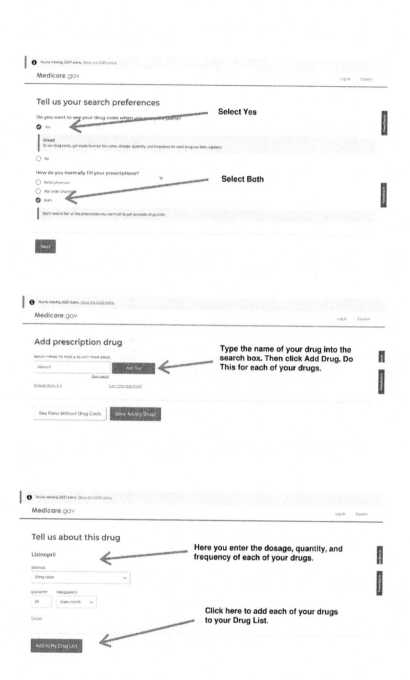

Select Yes

Select Both

Type the name of your drug into the search box. Then click Add Drug. Do This for each of your drugs.

Here you enter the dosage, quantity, and frequency of each of your drugs.

Click here to add each of your drugs to your Drug List.

55

Click here when you have added each of your drugs and you are ready to go to the next step.

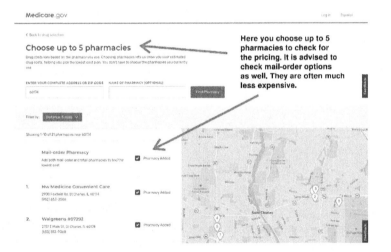

Here you choose up to 5 pharmacies to check for the pricing. It is advised to check mail-order options as well. They are often much less expensive.

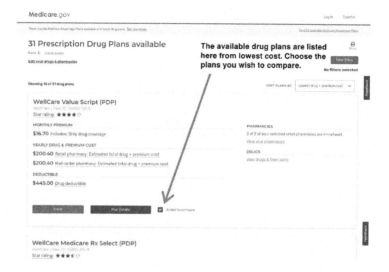

31 Prescription Drug Plans available

The available drug plans are listed here from lowest cost. Choose the plans you wish to compare.

WellCare Value Script (PDP)

WellCare Medicare Rx Select (PDP)

If you were successful in following the directions, the least expensive Prescription Drug Plan (PDP) will be at the top of the list.

Click "Add to Compare" on the first few plans and then click "COMPARE". On the next screen, up to three PDP plans will be listed side-by-side for your perusal.

This last comparison screen will show the final results of your plan search. Below the name of each plan you selected to compare, the total annual cost of prescriptions + insurance premiums is listed for each pharmacy that you chose early in the process.

Select the lowest cost plan you care to use based on your projected total annual cost at one or more of your favorite pharmacies.

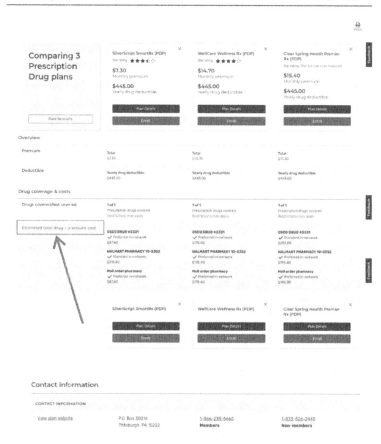

Choose the plan you prefer and click "Enroll" at the bottom. You may be able to enroll online. If you choose to telephone, call the "non-member" number.

Consider repeating this process next year at the Annual Enrollment Period (AEP) in the fall to ensure you have the lowest cost plan.

CHAPTER 12

What Will All of This Cost?

There is a monetary cost for all insurance coverage and government supplied health insurance is no exception. The good news is that, if you are coming off an Obamacare type of plan, the new costs will look like a bargain to you!

A note about IRMAA – the success penalty. This stands for Income Related Monthly Adjustment Amount and may add to the monthly premium for Medicare Part B and for the Prescription Drug Plan, based on what the IRS has recorded as your MAGI (Modified Adjusted Gross Income) two years ago.

The target audience for this book is likely to encounter the following monthly premium costs in 2021:

Medicare Part A

Free of Charge (after 40 quarters of taxable earnings)

Medicare Part B

$148.50 (IRMAA could increase it substantially)

Medicare Supplement Plans: Premiums vary widely depending on several factors. These include state of residence, age, sex, ZIP Code and sometimes smoking status, height & weight.

HIGH DEDUCTIBLE (high value) PLANS F or G -

Most cost effective – estimated between $30 and $80

PLAN F –

Most comprehensive -estimated between $140 & $250

PLAN G -

Lower priced than Plan F but Part B deductible ($203) is not covered

PDP –

Prescription Drug Plans - $7.00 and up, depending on plan and location plus drug deductibles, co-pay and co-insurance.

PDP premiums are also subject to an IRMAA penalty assessment.

2021 MEDICARE COST SHARING PROVISIONS

PART A - Deductible and co-insurance payable by you or your Supplement

Deductible per hospital admission = You pay $1,484

Co-insurance hospital days 1 to 60 = You pay $0

Co-insurance days 61 to 90 = You pay $371 per day

Co-insurance days 91 to 150 = You pay $742 per day

Skilled Nursing Facility:

Co-insurance days 0 to 20 = You pay $0

Co-insurance days 21 to 100 = You pay $185.50/day

PART B – Deductible and co-insurance payable by you or your Supplement

Annual Deductible = $203

Co-insurance (no limit) = 20%

IRMMA 2021- Part B (top) & Part D

The standard Part B premium amount in 2021 is $148.50. Most people pay the standard Part B premium amount. If your modified adjusted gross income as reported on your IRS tax return from 2 years ago is above a certain amount, you'll pay the standard premium amount and an Income Related Monthly Adjustment Amount (IRMAA). IRMAA is an extra charge added to your premium.

If your yearly income in 2019 (for what you pay in 2021) was

File individual tax return	File joint tax return	File married & separate tax return	You pay each month (in 2021)
$88,000 or less	$176,000 or less	$88,000 or less	$148.50
above $88,000 up to $111,000	above $176,000 up to $222,000	Not applicable	$207.90
above $111,000 up to $138,000	above $222,000 up to $276,000	Not applicable	$297.00
above $138,000 up to $165,000	above $276,000 up to $330,000	Not applicable	$386.10
above $165,000 and less than $500,000	above $330,000 and less than $750,000	above $88,000 and less than $412,000	$475.20
$500,000 or above	$750,000 and above	$412,000 and above	$504.90

If your filing status and yearly income in 2019 was

File individual tax return	File joint tax return	File married & separate tax return	You pay each month (in 2021)
$88,000 or less	$176,000 or less	$88,000 or less	your plan premium
above $88,000 up to $111,000	above $176,000 up to $222,000	not applicable	$12.30 + your plan premium
above $111,000 up to $138,000	above $222,000 up to $276,000	not applicable	$31.80 + your plan premium
above $138,000 up to $165,000	above $276,000 up to $330,000	not applicable	$51.20 + your plan premium
above $165,000 and less than $500,000	above $330,000 and less than $750,000	above $88,000 and less than $412,000	$70.70 + your plan premium
$500,000 or above	$750,000 and above	$412,000 and above	$77.10 + your plan premium

CHAPTER 13

MASSACHUSETTS, MINNESOTA &
WISCONSIN

The three states addressed here somehow managed to persuade the Federal Government to grant waivers allowing them to create their own Medicare Supplement plans. All of the general characteristics that make supplements superior to Advantage plans still apply to these outliers. For example, they work anywhere in the United States and they have no restrictive doctor or hospital networks.

Otherwise, the benefit structure of these state designed plans differs markedly from the Medicare Supplement plans we have discussed that are available in the other 47. The following descriptions are drawn, in part, from www.medicare.gov. To peruse the actual coverage details, go to that site and search "Medigap-in-(state)".

MASSACHUSETTS

 The Bay State has three plans available. One may buy the Core Plan or either Supplement 1 (only for those born before 1955) or Supplement 1A. Each of them includes the same set of Basic Benefits.

Each supplement has additional elements that fill the gaps in Original Medicare plus some state mandated benefits. The bottom line is that the Core Plan is lean and probably much less costly as a stand-alone rather than buying a supplement.

Want to save money? Obviously, the Core Plan is going to be less expensive than a Supplement Plan, no matter which insurance company is offering them. The only strategy I can see is to carefully examine the additional benefits covered by the Supplement 1 or 1A Plans to decide for yourself if the savings in premium dollars by purchasing only the Core Plan would be worth the risk.

As an example, you may not plan to travel abroad, or you have no expectation of being committed to a mental hospital. These are coverages you likely can avoid paying for without concern. However, you would want to think carefully about savings vs. risk of going without coverage for the Part A hospital deductible or the skilled nursing facility coinsurance.

Compare these plans side-by-side

If a "yes" appears, the plan covers the described benefit 100%. If "no" appears, the policy doesn't cover that benefit.

Medigap Benefits	Medigap Plans		
	Core Plan	Supplement 1	Supplement 1A
Basic benefits	Yes	Yes	Yes
Part A: inpatient hospital deductible	No	Yes	Yes
Part A: skilled nursing facility coinsurance	No	Yes	Yes
Part B: deductible*	No	Yes*	No
Foreign travel emergency	No	Yes	Yes
Inpatient days in mental health hospitals	60 days per calendar year	120 days per benefit year	120 days per benefit year
State-mandated benefits (yearly Pap tests and mammograms. Check your plan for other state-mandated benefits.)	No	Yes	Yes

MINNESOTA

In the North Star State there is a plethora of Medicare Supplement plans available for sale.

The Basic and Extended Basic plans are described in the chart below. They are available when you enroll in Part B, regardless of your age or health problems.

Compare these plans side-by-side

If a "yes" appears, the plan covers the described benefit 100%. If a row lists a percentage, the policy covers that percentage of the described benefit. If a "no" appears, the policy doesn't cover that benefit.

Medigap Benefits	Medigap Plans	
	Basic Plan	Extended Basic Plan
Basic benefits	Yes	Yes
Part A: inpatient hospital deductible	No	Yes
Part A: skilled nursing facility coinsurance	Yes (Provides 100 days of SNF care)	Yes (Provides 120 days of SNF care)
Part B: deductible**	No	Yes**
Foreign travel emergency	80%	80%'
Outpatient mental health	50%	50%
Usual and customary fees	No	80%'
Medicare-cover preventative care	Yes	Yes
Physical therapy	20%	20%
Coverage while in a foreign country	No	80%'
State-mandated benefits (diabetic equipment and supplies, routine cancer screening, reconstructive surgery, and immunizations)	Yes	Yes

Insurance companies may offer 4 additional riders that can be added to a Basic Plan. You may choose any or all of these riders to design a policy that meets your needs:

1) Part A deductible
2) Part B deductible (only for those eligible for Medicare but not enrolled before 2020)
3) Usual and customary fees
4) Non-Medicare preventive care

Minnesota versions of Medicare Supplement plans K, L, M, N plus High Deductible Plan F (for those born before 1955) are also available.

If old enough I would take a close look at High Deductible Plan F. Otherwise, some careful shopping and comparisons will be necessary.

WISCONSIN

 The Badger State has taken a build-your-own approach to Medicare Supplement coverage.

Of course, there are the ever-present Basic Benefits but they are included in the Basic Plan which also covers:

1) Part A: skilled nursing facility coinsurance
2) 175 days per lifetime in addition to Medicare's benefit of inpatient mental health coverage
3) 40 additional home health care visits
4) State mandated benefits

Insurance companies are also allowed to offer these riders:

- Part A deductible
- 365 additional home health care visits
- Part B deductible
- Part B excess charges
- Foreign travel emergency
- 50% Part A deductible
- Part B copayment or coinsurance

There is also a High Deductible, **high value plan** available with a $2370 deductible.

If I were shopping for a Medicare Supplement in Wisconsin, that high value plan would be the first thing I would look at.

CHAPTER 14
The only chapter you are likely to need!

Are you in charge of your own health insurance and hoping to simplify the Medicare coverage selection process?

The next few pages will allow you to ignore the prevailing confusion and purchase the best, most comprehensive medical insurance available.

STEP 1.

Have you selected your Medicare Part A start date? (Read more in Chapter 3)

Have you selected your Medicare Part B start date? (Read more in Chapter 4)

ENROLL IN MEDICARE ONLINE HERE:

https://www.ssa.gov/medicare/

Scroll down to find the blue button that says:

Apply for Medicare Only

The enrollment process could take as little as 10 minutes.

Only two more steps to go!

STEP 2.

Decide on and apply for your Medicare supplement plan.

For this step you need a licensed insurance agent.

If you would like me to act as your agent, go to:

www.MedicareForTheLazyMan.com

Scroll to the US map and click your state.
A very short questionnaire will appear that you can send to me and we will begin the process.

What follows are descriptions of the two types of Medicare supplement plans I recommend and sell:

CHOOSE YOUR MEDICARE SUPPLEMENT PLAN

LUXURIOUS CADILLAC OF MEDICARE SUPPLEMENT PLANS – most comprehensive coverage. Best suited for those with comfortable finances, low risk tolerance and desiring 100% coverage no matter the cost.

PLAN F: Formerly the most popular choice and only available to those born before 1955. This has generally the highest monthly premium but has the richest benefit structure. PLAN F pays 100% of all deductibles, co-pays and co-insurance. The insured will not receive any invoices for cost sharing expenses when all medical treatment is Medicare approved.

Unfortunately, my observation is that insurance companies are raising the rates on Plan F drastically.

PLAN G: Set to become the most popular choice and certainly the richest benefit structure after PLAN F. Pays all of the expenses listed above except for the annual $203 Part B annual deductible. This is the simplest and richest plan available to those first becoming eligible for Medicare in 2020 or later.

HIGH PERFORMANCE PONTIAC GTO OF MEDICARE SUPPLEMENT PLANS – most cost-effective coverage

Best suited for those having somewhat higher risk tolerance, willing to accept some limited cost sharing expenses in return for a substantially lower monthly premium cost.

HIGH DEDUCTIBLE PLAN F: Covers all of the risks of legitimate expenses as are covered by PLAN F above. However, instead of paying at 100% from day one of each year, it pays at something less than 100% with the insured making up the relatively small difference. In the unlikely event of very high medical expenses, the plan starts paying 100% after the insured's portion adds up to $2,370 (in 2021). Substantially lower monthly premium than PLAN F, but is not available to those born in 1955 or later.

HIGH DEDUCTIBLE PLAN G: Protects just like HDF above except does not credit the $203 Part B annual deductible. If the $2,370 plan deductible is reached during a period of unusual medical expenses, it will pay 100% for the balance of the year just as its big brother Plan G would.

READ MORE ABOUT MEDICARE SUPPLEMENT PLANS
IN CHAPTERS 6, 7, & 8

STEP 3.

Select the least expensive Prescription Drug Plan (PDP)

from a list of all plans available in your area.

Purchase that plan online directly from the insurance company.

In Chapter 11 you will find step-by-step navigation instructions leading you to that list of PDP plans arranged in order of annual cost.

These instructions look complicated, but it is a government website and so was not designed to be user-friendly. The most complicated part of the process will be entering the detail for each of your current prescription medications.

Since the PDPs are one-year contracts, annual costs can change at the discretion of each insurance company. Also, your prescription drug needs may change during the course of the year.

Therefore, you may find this a worthwhile project to do each year during the Annual Election Period (AEP) in the fall, in case you would like to buy a new plan for the following year.

<u>EASY NAVIGATION INSTRUCTIONS TO SELECT AND PURCHASE A LOW-COST PDP:</u>

THE STEPS ARE ILLUSTRATED IN CHAPTER 11!

If you were successful, CONGRATULATIONS! Your Medicare prescription drug plan (PDP) work is done!

Furthermore, if you were able to complete all three of these steps, you now have acquired the four essential elements of protection:

MEDICARE PART A

MEDICARE PART B

MEDICARE SUPPLEMENT PLANS

PRESCRIPTION DRUG PLANS

CHAPTER 15

Did You Make A Boo-Boo?

It is very likely that you are hearing about the excellent benefits of Medicare supplement plans and especially the great cost advantage of High Deductible **"High Value"** PLANS F & G (HDF and HDG) for the first time.

Since commissions payable to agents are more substantial for Medicare Advantage plans, those are the ones that are promoted most vigorously to the unsuspecting public.

Is that the case with you?

Were you kept in the dark about Medicare supplements and High Deductible, **"High Value"** plans?

Are you anxious to make a change so that you can enjoy the benefits of Medicare supplement plans along with all of my happy clients?

Well, I have good news and bad news for you:

GOOD NEWS: You may apply for a Medicare supplement policy from an insurance carrier any time the mood strikes!

BAD NEWS: There is no "guaranteed issue" period for Medicare supplement plans after your initial enrollment period when you first became eligible. You MAY be asked a series of questions about your medical history in order to prove that you are insurable.

This is not true in every instance or in every state but generally you will have to jump through some hoops in order to be allowed to buy a Medicare supplement policy outside of the initial enrollment period. You might be refused if your medical condition and history do not meet the insurance company's insurability standards.

There are a few special exceptions but understanding them and the related complexities is what makes Medicare so much fun.

I may be able to help, and I would like to try!

CONTACT ME:

DBJ@MLMmailbag.com

www.MedicareForTheLazyMan.com

ACKNOWLEDGMENTS

This book would not exist. I would still be sitting at my desk with fingers poised over the keys and eyes caressing the mountains around our Arizona home were it not for my wife.

Mary is among my most rabid critics but can often be brought around to my way of thinking with some persistent persuasion. Once on my team, she is an invaluable asset and a source of insight, inspiration, motivation and support.

Mary is not really high maintenance, but she does need to be reminded periodically that "spousal unit" is actually a term of loving endearment. Not much else to say after almost 50 years of partnership and teamwork.

Thanks to my personal clients who helped me form the idea for this project after realizing why they were all so frustrated.

Others, generally without being pestered, have explained complicated technological mysteries, prodded me out of lethargy or sharpened red pencils to gleefully perform surgery on my sterling prose.

They have shared companionship, cocktails, encouragement, ribald jokes and philosophical pontification, all without ever a negative word about this relatively ambitious project. So I also thank, in no particular order:

Randy & Margaret Carson of C2C Consulting, LLC

Brian and Teri Jones   Tony and Melisa Coletto

Gerry and Lisa Schafer   Roy & Kathy Brotherhood

Paul and Kathleen Bowling

Finally, for no reason other than I just enjoy them, I must acknowledge the youngest generation of my gene pool. Thanks for making the rest of us proud and happy to have you in our family:

Max Coletto & Alex Coletto - Californians just starting to spread their wings.

Drew and Magda McMillin, Robbie McMillin and Kate McMillin –

Canadian-Americans proud to wave both flags!

ABOUT THE AUTHOR

Douglas B. Jones, CLU, RHU

Medicare snuck up on me just as it does with most Americans.

As a long-time health insurance professional, I was expected by friends and clients to be ahead of the curve. Turns out I needed to educate myself on this complex subject in order to be able to offer solid advice.

After graduation from the University of Arizona I joined my family's John Hancock insurance agency in Chicago's Loop. Even though life insurance sales with the John Hancock was a 3-generation family calling, I found more satisfaction in helping clients with their health insurance needs.

Eventually the company stopped offering those products so I left to pursue my mission with other companies.

Decades later at a social event, I was asked by several people for a short version of my Medicare advice. They assumed I must be an expert since we were all rapidly approaching age 65.

That was the catalyst that convinced me to learn what Medicare was all about. After a period of study, I formed some conclusions that are directly at odds with other Medicare advisors.

One evening a couple of longtime friends came over to act as my Guinea pigs. The wife, ever the serious student, was lugging all of the printed material they had received and expected me to educate them on every one of the Medicare options available in our area.

The husband was mostly interested in the beer I offered. His opinion was that this whole Medicare decision process was an unpleasant inconvenience that should end quickly.

Very soon, these friends had a complete grasp of my best Medicare advice and the reasons behind it. They were stunned that the whole thing could be boiled down to such a simple conclusion. As they discovered, the most time-consuming part of the process was completing the insurance paperwork.

That evening set the pattern for virtually all of my subsequent encounters with Medicare eligible citizens. Years later it occurred to me that the same process could be offered to everyone in the country who was staring down the barrel of Medicare.

Thus, was born Medicare for the Lazy Man!

Made in the USA
Middletown, DE
29 May 2021